Weight Loss Secret

15 tested tips

Written and translated
by Fabien BEAR

Table of contents

Preamble

My name is BEAR Fabien, and I have been a health and nutrition specialist coach for over 10 years. I have worked with many clients who are looking to lose weight, and I have seen how challenging it can be for some people. That's why I decided to write this book to share my knowledge and tips with a wider audience.

I wrote this book to help people who are looking to lose weight quickly and effectively. I know that many people have tried different diets and exercise programs without success, and I wanted to provide practical and proven tips to help them achieve their weight loss goals.

My goal is to provide realistic and sustainable advice that can help people lose weight in a healthy and balanced way.
This book is designed to be easy to use and navigate. You can read each chapter in order or focus on the sections that interest you the most.

In each chapter, you will find practical tips, advice, and information about weight loss. I encourage you to take notes and use these tips in your daily life to help you achieve your weight loss goals.

Introduction

Losing weight may seem challenging, but it is an achievable goal that can significantly improve your health and quality of life. Excess weight can increase the risk of chronic diseases such as diabetes, heart disease, and high blood pressure. In addition, weight loss can increase self-esteem and improve self-image.

In this book, we will present 15 simple and practical tips to help you lose weight in a healthy and effective way. These tips are based on scientific research and have been tested by many people. They are intended to be easy to implement and adaptable to different lifestyles.

Before starting, it is important to note that each person is different, and results may vary. It is also essential to consult a healthcare professional before starting any diet or exercise program.

How to Use This Book to Achieve Your Weight Loss Goals

This book is designed to help you lose weight in a healthy and effective way. You can use this book in different ways, depending on your needs and preferences. You can browse the entire book to familiarize yourself with the different tips, or you can focus on the tips that work best for you.

You can also use this book as a reference guide by regularly revisiting the tips that have helped you lose weight. Each tip will be presented in detail, with practical advice to help you implement them into your daily life.

By following the tips presented in this book, you can not only lose weight but also improve your overall health and quality of life. We hope this book will be useful to you on your journey towards a healthier and happier life.

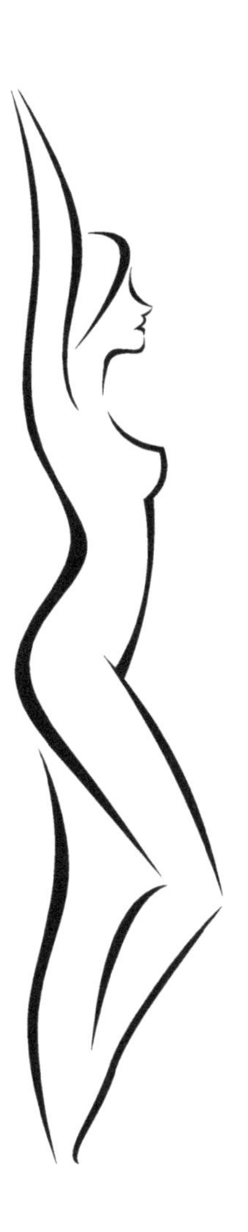

Understanding weight loss

Losing weight may seem complex, but in reality, it is based on relatively simple basic principles. In this chapter, we will explore the fundamental principles of weight loss so that you can better understand how it works and how you can apply it to your life.

The Basic Principles of Weight Loss

Weight loss is dependent on energy balance, which is the balance between the calories you consume and the calories you burn. If you consume more calories than you burn, you will gain weight. If you burn more calories than you consume, you will lose weight.

To lose weight effectively, you need to create a calorie deficit by burning more calories than you consume. This can be accomplished by reducing the amount of calories you consume, increasing the amount of calories you burn through exercise, or a combination of both.

However, it is important to note that healthy and sustainable weight loss is not just about reducing calories. It is also important to follow a balanced diet and exercise regularly. Healthy food choices and exercise can help improve overall health, increase metabolism, and burn fat.

Furthermore, it is important to understand that weight loss does not happen overnight. It requires patience, perseverance, and sustained effort. Keeping this in mind, we will explore practical and effective tips in the following chapters to help you lose weight in a healthy and sustainable way.

15 Tips

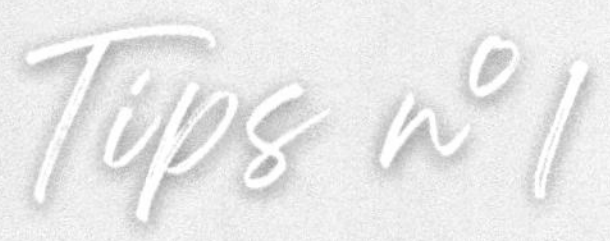

Start your day with a healthy breakfast

Breakfast is often considered the **most important meal** of the day.

Indeed, it can help **boost metabolism, control appetite, and provide the energy** needed to start the day off right.

For a healthy breakfast, choose foods that are rich in protein, fiber, and nutrients, such as eggs, fruits, vegetables, and whole grains.

Drink water throughout the day

Drinking enough water is essential for maintaining good hydration and helping to **regulate appetite**.

In fact, dehydration can often be **confused with hunger, which can lead to overeating**.

For optimal hydration, drink water throughout the day and avoid sugary and alcoholic beverages.

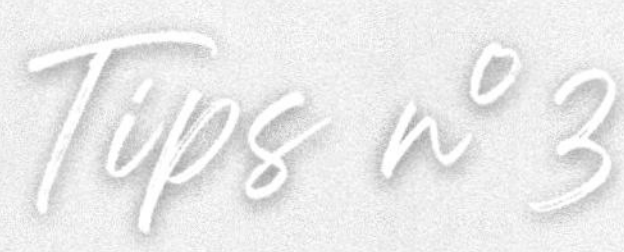

Avoid processed foods and those high in sugar

Processed foods and those high in sugar can contribute to **excessive weight gain.**

In fact, they are often high in calories, added sugars, and unhealthy fats.

For a healthy diet, choose **whole and fresh foods** such as fruits, vegetables, lean meats, and whole grains.

Eat fiber-rich foods

Fiber-rich foods can help **regulate appetite, maintain stable blood sugar levels, and improve digestion.**

For a high-fiber diet, choose foods such as fruits, vegetables, nuts and seeds, legumes, and whole grains.

Limit your intake of saturated fats

Saturated fats can contribute to excessive weight gain and health problems such as heart disease.

For a healthy diet, limit your intake of saturated fats by **choosing low-fat foods**, such as **lean meats, reduced-fat dairy products, and healthy vegetable oils.**

Plan your meals

Meal planning can help you avoid **unhealthy food choices** and **maintain a balanced diet.**

To plan your meals, take the time to **make a grocery list, prepare meals in advance, and choose healthy and tasty foods for each meal**.

By applying these tips for a healthy diet, you will be on the right track to reaching your goals.

Choose lean proteins

Proteins are essential for **building muscles and recovery**, which is important when you are active.

Foods rich in lean proteins include fish, poultry, tofu, legumes, and low-fat dairy products.

Choosing lean proteins can help **reduce the risk of cardiovascular disease, high blood pressure, type 2 diabetes, and obesity.**

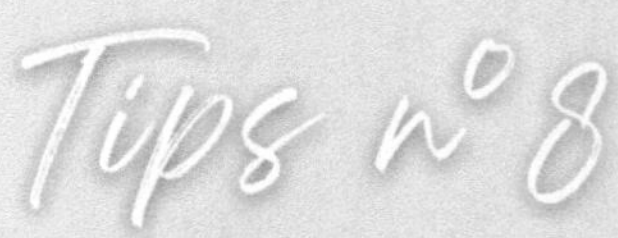

Avoid skipping meals or starving yourself

Skipping meals or depriving yourself of food can **slow down your metabolism** and lead to cravings.

To maintain a balanced diet, regularly eat healthy and nourishing meals.

Find a **balance** between eating enough food to meet your needs while choosing healthy foods.

Exercise regularly.

Regular exercise is essential for **healthy and sustainable weight loss**.

Exercise can help **burn calories, increase metabolism, and strengthen muscle mass.**

To lose weight, it is recommended to do at least 150 to 300 minutes of moderate-intensity exercise or 75 to 150 minutes of vigorous-intensity exercise per week.

Find ways to manage your stress

Stress can **stimulate appetite** and **encourage fat storage**, which can hinder weight loss.

To manage stress, find strategies that work for you, such as **meditation, yoga, physical exercise, or therapy.**

Take the time to do activities you enjoy and spend time with positive and supportive people.

Get enough sleep each night

Getting enough sleep each night can help **regulate appetite and metabolism**, thus promoting weight loss.

It is recommended to sleep between 7 and 9 hours each night. Create a **consistent sleep routine** and avoid stimulants before bed to maximize the benefits of sleep on your diet.

Utilize food and exercise tracking tools.

Food and exercise tracking tools can help you become more aware of **what you eat and your level of activity.**

This can assist you in **adjusting your diet** and **exercise regimen** to more effectively achieve your weight loss goals.

Find a friend or family member to support you

Find someone who **shares** your weight loss goal and can help you stay motivated.

You can **exercise together, cook healthy meals together,** or simply **support** each other when needed.

Reward yourself with non-food items

Instead of rewarding yourself with food, find ways to reward yourself that are not food-related.

For example, treat yourself to a **massage** or a **new outfit** when you reach a weight loss goal.

Be patient and realistic in your weight loss expectations

Losing weight can take time.

Be **patient** and **realistic** in your expectations.

Set achievable **goals** and celebrate every small success along the way

Weight loss may seem like a daunting task, but with the tips provided in this book, you can realistically and healthily achieve your goals. In summary, key weight loss tips include healthy dietary changes, regular physical activity, additional support, and personal motivation.

It's also important to remember that weight loss is not a quick fix, but an ongoing process that requires patience and determination. You can maintain your weight loss by adopting a healthy lifestyle and using food and exercise tracking tools to sustain your eating and fitness habits.

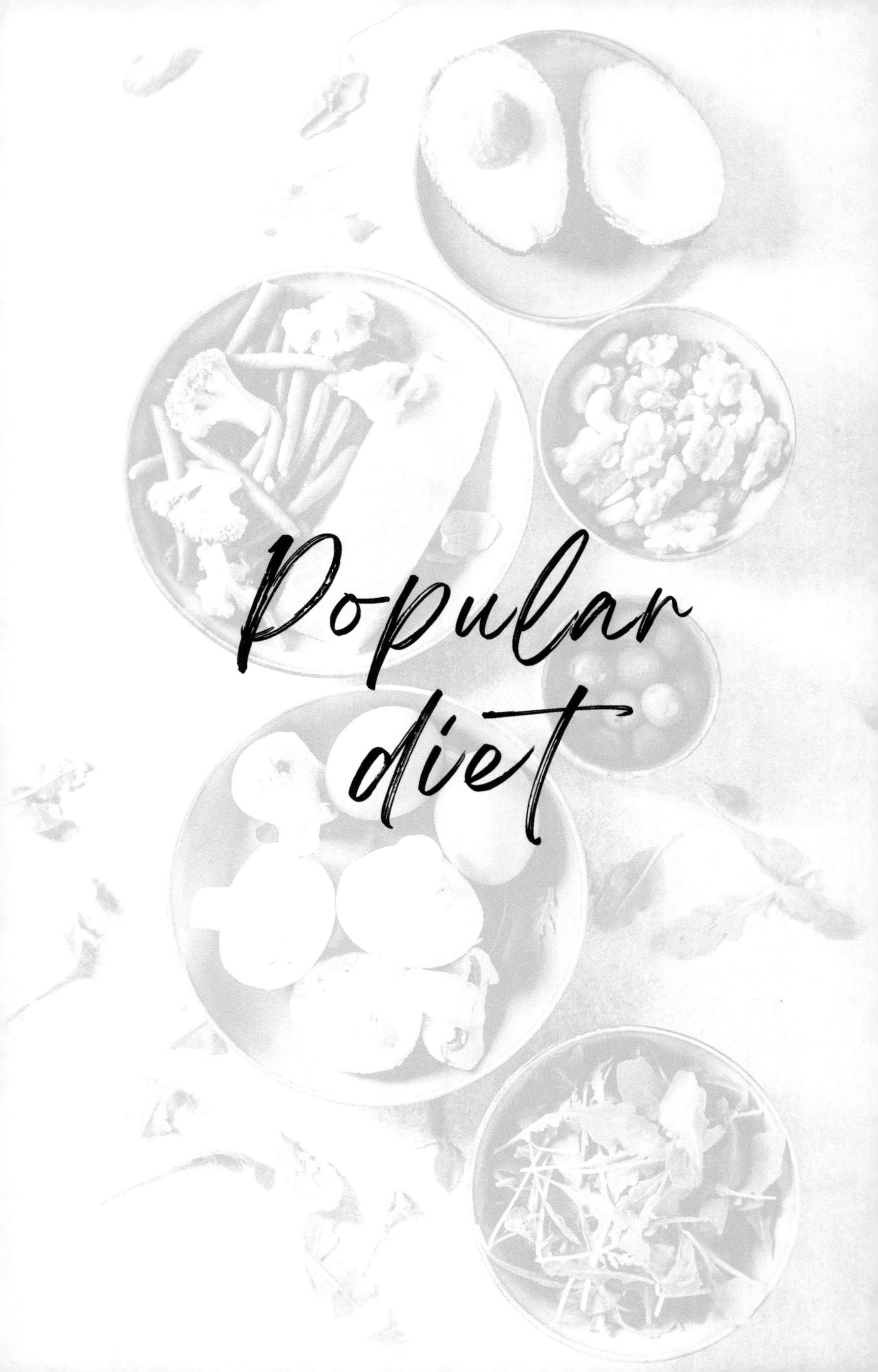
Popular
diet

In this section, we will examine some of the most popular diets for quick weight loss. It's important to note that every individual is different and what works for one person may not work for another. Before starting a new diet, it's important to consult with your doctor or healthcare professional to ensure that it's safe and appropriate for you.

Keto diet

The ketogenic (or keto) diet is a low-carb, high-fat diet that aims to train your body to burn fat for energy instead of carbohydrates. This diet involves consuming about 70 to 80% of your calories in the form of fats, 20 to 25% in the form of proteins, and only 5 to 10% in the form of carbohydrates.

The ketogenic diet was initially developed to treat epilepsy in children, but it is now becoming increasingly popular for weight loss. By limiting carbohydrates, the body enters a state of ketosis, where it begins to use stored fats in the body as a source of energy. Foods commonly consumed in a ketogenic diet include meats, avocados, nuts, seeds, low-carb vegetables, and healthy fats such as olive oil and coconut oil.

However, it is important to note that this diet is not for everyone and may require close medical monitoring to avoid undesirable side effects such as fatigue, headaches, and constipation.

Paleo diet

The Paleo (or Paleolithic) diet aims to mimic the diet of our hunter-gatherer ancestors by avoiding processed foods and focusing on whole foods such as meats, vegetables, and fruits. This diet eliminates processed foods, sugar, grains, and legumes.

The Paleo diet is based on the assumption that our bodies have not evolved to process processed foods, refined sugars, and modern grains, leading to health problems such as obesity and heart disease. The diet encourages the consumption of unprocessed whole foods such as lean meats, green vegetables, fruits, nuts, and seeds, as these foods provide essential nutrients such as protein, healthy fats, and fiber. However, it is important to note that the Paleo diet can be expensive and restrictive, and it can be difficult to follow such a strict diet in the long term.

Vegetarian diet

The vegetarian diet is a diet that excludes meat, fish, and seafood, but may include dairy products and eggs. This diet can help reduce the consumption of saturated fats and cholesterol, but it is important to ensure that enough protein and essential nutrients are obtained.

The vegetarian diet can be beneficial for health as it is often rich in fiber, vitamins, minerals, and antioxidants. However, it is important for vegetarians to ensure they get enough protein, iron, calcium, and vitamin B12, which are nutrients commonly found in meat. Vegetarian sources of protein include legumes, nuts, seeds, dairy products, and eggs.

Vegetarians should also be aware of processed carbohydrate-rich foods, similar to non-vegetarians. A well-planned vegetarian diet can be healthy and nutritious, but it is important to consult a healthcare professional to ensure that your nutritional needs are met.

Gluten free diet

The gluten-free diet involves avoiding foods that contain gluten, a protein found in grains such as wheat, barley, and rye. This diet is often used for people with celiac disease, who are intolerant to gluten, but some people also choose to follow this diet for weight loss.

The gluten-free diet can help people with celiac disease avoid symptoms associated with gluten intolerance, such as abdominal pain, diarrhea, and fatigue. However, it is important to note that simply avoiding gluten does not guarantee weight loss. In fact, many gluten-free foods, such as gluten-free baked goods, can be high in calories, sugar, and fat. To lose weight while following a gluten-free diet, it is important to focus on whole and healthy foods such as fruits, vegetables, lean meats, nuts, and seeds.

It is important to note that all of these diets have their advantages and disadvantages, and what works for one person may not work for another. It is important to discuss any new dietary approach with a healthcare professional.

Physical exercises

Physical exercise is an important element of any weight loss strategy. In this section, we will examine the most effective types of exercises for burning calories and losing weight, as well as tips for planning your exercise program.

Cardiovascular exercices

Cardiovascular exercises are beneficial for heart health, weight loss, and building endurance. They increase your heart rate, which increases the amount of oxygen transported throughout your body. When your body uses more oxygen, it burns more calories and fats, which helps to reduce weight and body fat. Cardiovascular exercises are also useful for improving your blood circulation, strengthening your immune system, reducing stress, and improving your mood. Additionally, these types of exercises can be practiced in many different ways, making them accessible to a wide range of people, regardless of their level of fitness.

Strength training exercises

Strength training exercises, such as free weights, weight machines, and resistance bands, are exercises that strengthen and tone your muscles.

Although strength training exercises do not burn as many calories as cardiovascular exercises, they can help increase your metabolism and burn fat in the long term.

Strength training exercises can increase your muscle mass, which increases the amount of calories you burn even at rest. This means that you will continue to burn fat even after your workout. Strength training exercises can also improve your posture, strengthen your bones, and reduce the risk of injury. It is recommended to combine strength training exercises with cardiovascular exercises to achieve the best results in terms of weight loss and overall health.

How to plan your exercise program

Pour perdre du poids, vous devez brûler plus de calories que vous n'en consommez. La quantité d'exercice dont vous avez besoin dépend de votre niveau de forme physique et de vos objectifs de perte de poids.

Voici quelques conseils pour planifier votre programme d'exercice :

Commencez lentement : Si vous êtes nouveau dans l'exercice, commencez lentement et augmentez progressivement l'intensité et la durée de vos séances d'entraînement.

Vary your workout sessions: Alternate between cardiovascular exercises and strength training exercises to burn calories and strengthen your muscles.

Find activities you enjoy: Choose activities you enjoy, such as dancing or hiking, to motivate you to exercise regularly.

Set realistic goals: Set realistic weight loss goals and track your progress using an exercise journal or fitness tracking app.

Stay consistent: Plan your exercise program and try to stick to it as much as possible.

Conclusion

In this book, we have covered several aspects of weight loss and how to lose weight quickly and effectively. We have discussed the basic principles of weight loss and different types of diets. We have also shared many tips for eating less, burning more calories, and staying motivated throughout your weight loss journey. We have also covered cardiovascular exercises and strength training exercises as well as tips on how to plan your exercise program.

In conclusion, weight loss is a process that can be challenging, but with the right tools and strategies, you can succeed. We hope this book has provided you with helpful tips to help you lose weight quickly and effectively.

Remember that it's important to avoid common mistakes and maintain your weight loss long-term. If you need additional help, don't hesitate to seek the assistance of a healthcare professional or coach.

Thanks !